HOW TO LOSE BODY FAT AND MAINTAIN YOUR WEIGHT

LOSE KILOS WITHOUT REBOUND EFFECT, ELIMINATE ABDOMINAL AND LEG FAT, BURN CALORIES QUICKLY IN A NATURAL WAY

Jessy M. Brown

First Edition

Table of Contents

Introduction...4

The Reality of Weight Loss.....................................6

How to control body weight?.....................9

Fashion diets..13

All about exercises.......................................17

The role of emotions in weight loss...................21

How to set objectives?.................................25

Learning to eat... 29

Alternatives to Weight Loss......................33

Conclusion..37

Introduction

Losing weight cannot be achieved in the blink of an eye. Before you reach your ultimate goal, you have to take precise steps and get rid of your unhealthy lifestyle. Depending on your preferred schemes, losing weight can be easy or complicated.

Weight loss requires a reduction in calorie intake. Most people try to lose weight through exercise or diet.

Each person has their own reason for choosing to lose weight. Some of them want to develop their self-confidence or look more attractive, while others just want to stay healthy and fit. Whatever reasons you have, there's nothing to worry about. Achieving a perfect body and weight can be done without practicing any complicated procedures. It's about how you control yourself and motivate yourself to live a healthy lifestyle.

To learn more about weight loss and maintenance, this book will serve as your definitive guide. Through this, you have the opportunity to recognize your fundamental facts. So start reading this book and start improving your weight condition and lifestyle.

The Reality of Weight Loss

Whether you want to stay in shape, change your body to a perfect one or look sexier, you have to understand the whole concept of weight loss. If you read health news regularly, you'll probably recognize that the rate of obesity tends to increase. This alarming condition has awakened health professionals and organizations. As a result, they are providing appropriate advice and solutions to solve this problem. However, the help of these health agencies is not enough.

If you really want to reduce your weight, you have to help yourself. You need to be more aware of your lifestyle and daily activities.

Weight loss refers to a reduction in total body mass characterized by a loss of skeletal muscle and body fat. This term comes in two types:

- Intentional weight loss - When a person intentionally reduces their weight, they often plan a diet or training program. These programs are designed to lose a certain amount of weight in a short period of time.

- Unintentional weight loss - Weight loss can be accidental if a person is suffering from any untreated health problem. Typical examples of this are diabetes, stress, anxiety and much more.

As experts say, losing weight offers multiple benefits. In addition to an impressive appearance, you also have the opportunity to live for more years. Obese people often suffer from multiple diseases such as diabetes, hypertension, heart disease and cancer.

> ➢ *Weight Loss Considerations and Tips*

Even if you choose to lose weight

instantly, it is essential to avoid shock diets, fad diets, frequent fasting, and other measures of intense weight loss. These plans can put you at risk for health problems.

For example, people who use laxatives while dieting may develop dehydration, kidney problems, heart problems, and intestinal damage.

The best way to lose more weight is to eat a diet that covers the right healthy foods. This can help maintain body function while reducing weight. Before doing any activity or participating in any program, be sure to consult with your nutritionist or physician.

When making a weight loss plan, you should always include proper exercise. In addition to burning calories through intense physical activity, regular training develops a resting metabolism. Therefore, it can help the body burn more calories while doing ordinary activities.

How to control body weight?

Not everyone knows how to lose weight. Sometimes, they just rely on several programs that aim to reduce more body fat and achieve a perfect figure. Before you start reducing your fat, you must first understand the fundamental facts of weight management.

Weight management is defined as a lasting approach to a healthy lifestyle. It encompasses a balance between physical exercise and healthy eating to link energy intake and energy expenditure. Understanding your body's needs is essential to weight management. It can also control over- or underconsumption of food.

Nutritionists claim that weight management does not cover fad diets. It often focuses on the long-term outcomes followed by maintaining body weight. If you control your weight, you can achieve not only a perfect figure, but also prevent chronic diseases.

> ## *Weight control methods*

Weight management comes in multiple methods. Some are easy to follow, while others need constant monitoring and strict enforcement. For more details about these schemes, here are some of their various methods that you should know:

- More protein intake - Food specialists say that protein intake at breakfast has a greater effect compared to subsequent meals. It also has a greater thermogenic effect than fats and carbohydrates. If you eat protein-rich foods at breakfast, this helps increase glucagon activity.

- Use smaller plates - Through the use of smaller plates, it helps you consume smaller portions of food. Therefore, opportunities to consume fewer

calories are observed. If you continue to use larger dishes, you will always be tempted to consume larger portions and that leads to weight gain.

- Eating low-calorie foods - An average decrease in calorie intake always leads to slow weight loss. Lettuce, broccoli, grapefruit, cauliflower, and other low-calorie foods are recommended.

- Eat more dairy foods - Most nutritionists say consuming dairy products can reduce body fat. This happens because a greater amount of calcium in the diet develops the amount of energy and fat that is removed from the body.

- Stop drinking soda or sugary drinks - One of the main factors contributing to weight gain is sugary drinks. Even if these drinks are delicious and seem harmless, carbonated drinks consist of a large amount of calories. To avoid calories, you should always drink more water. Experts suggest consuming

eight to ten glasses of water regularly.

 - Sleeping Adequately - Since most people are busy doing their personal activities, they often neglect to practice proper sleep habits. If you sleep on time, it helps increase metabolism and relieves stress on the body. These aspects are related to weight loss and rapid metabolism.

 With your understanding of these schemes, you can make methods that will help reduce fat and maintain a healthy lifestyle.

Fashion diets

All people who want to reduce body fat are willing to try several diets that they have seen on popular television talk shows, magazines, or books. Most of these diets promise to provide perfect and quick results. Today, these diets are known as "fad diets". What are these fad diets and how effective are they?

Fad diets refer to any diet program or plan that claims to have discovered the latest secrets to losing weight. These diets are increasingly popular because they promise quick results, offer easy procedures, and are affordable.

Most fad diets are based on macronutrient manipulations. They consist of a low calorie intake to get their weight loss effects. In addition, they are not backed by rigorous scientific research and can be harmful to your health. Some fad diets restrict total energy intake. They also reduce carbohydrate intake for rapid weight loss.

The 3 fad diets that really work

If you're willing to practice fad diets, you need to know what kinds of diets work and what don't. For additional guidance, here are the three fad diets that really work:

1. Master Cleanse Diet Lemonade - Studies have shown that there are celebrities who practice this plan. This diet includes the exclusive consumption of lemonade cleanser based on lemons, water, maple syrup and cayenne pepper. Compared to other methods, it is quite difficult, since it is not necessary to eat any food.

2. Low-calorie, low-fat diets - This diet comes with a low calorie intake. It also leads to weight loss, but you need to follow strict methods. However, people on this diet need to control their daily food intake. If not, they can easily gain weight.

3. High-protein, low-carbohydrate diets - The best known high-protein, low-carbohydrate diet is the Atkins diet. Promotes the complete elimination of carbohydrates. Therefore, it offers rapid weight loss and a healthy body condition.

Some people believe that fad diets are quite harmful to their health. However, this is not always the case. It's simply how to choose the best fad diet available on the market. If you're planning to practice any fad diet, expect the following benefits:

- Motivation - The ultimate challenge of losing weight is staying motivated. If you change your exercise and eating habits, you need a big commitment. Sometimes, when you have noticed that the results are too slow, you may feel discouraged or frustrated. However, if you continue the process, you will notice that you are reducing more fat and have the perfect body you wanted.

  - Offers good health - Fad diets like raw diets eliminate all foods that are processed or cooked. They also focus on the consumption of fresh vegetables and fruits. The Atkins diet, on the other hand, helps reduce carbohydrate intake. The key to good health is to eat a variety of foods rich in vitamins and nutrients.

  - Awareness - A fad diet can make you feel active or energetic. Whatever type of fad diet you choose to practice, you should always be aware of the different foods you need to eat. You'll also know which foods are perfect for your body condition and which are not.

  With great information about these fad diets, you can easily decide which of them suits the needs of your healthy body condition. After finding the best diets, be sure to follow each step and be aware of your daily lifestyle.

All about exercises

Exercise and weight loss revolve around one word: calories. Although people need food to survive, there is always a limitation. Let us say, for example, that excessive consumption of carbohydrates is not advisable. To burn more fat, you need to do a couple of exercises. Whether you want a gentle or intense routine, you should always follow your procedures.

An ideal weight loss exercise includes a combination of weight training and aerobic exercise. Experts say that if you keep exercising every day, you're more likely to maintain your weight for longer and achieve a healthier body condition.

Because there are several weight-loss exercises, some of you may find it difficult to choose one. To solve this problem, here are the few training methods you should follow:

*- **Aerobic exercise** -*This is a type of exercise that develops breathing and heart rate over a continuous, sustained period. Typical examples of this exercise include swimming, bicycling, taking steps, and walking. For best results, you can do at least two or three exercises a day.

*- **Cardio exercises with equipment** -* Machines can offer multiple cardiovascular exercises. The most common examples are elliptical trainers, climbers, adaptive movement trainers and much more. Most of these devices help monitor your heart rate while reducing more body fat.

*- **Strength Training** -* This is perfect for all ages and recognized as a vital component of fitness. Whether you want to do weight lifting or weight-bearing exercises, you can help increase or maintain muscle mass. You can also reduce weight and develop a healthy body condition.

Apart from the above, there are several weight loss exercises. In fact, there are some people who prefer to enter several fitness gyms. For those who are quite busy, they prefer to do intense exercises at home.

As you continue to exercise, your heart rate tends to increase. As a result, your metabolism also develops and the chances of burning more fats are increasing greatly. For every minute of training, you can burn a specific amount of calories. The calories burned depend on how dynamic your exercise is. Studies have shown that the more calories you burn during exercise, the more calories you'll have. Therefore, you can lose more weight in a short period of time.

In addition, when you continue training, glucose is slowly depleted. The body then resorts to its fat storage and burns the internal fat to produce energy to replace the glucose. This means that when you burn more fat, you will lose weight will be

noticeable.

Even if there are multiple weight loss exercises, some still find it difficult to achieve their ultimate goal. If you are one of them, the best option you should take is to make a diary. In your diary, you have to write down your daily activities. You should also detail the different foods you need to eat while training. To make sure you follow your training plan, you have to encourage yourself. You can also list the many reasons why you choose to lose weight. In this way, you will always be inspired to carry out the necessary activities.

The role of emotions in weight loss

Believe it or not, your emotions play a vital role in your weight condition. Sometimes depressed people prefer to eat more food to relieve the feeling of discomfort. Others also turn to food for comfort, especially when they are stressed and frustrated by their work. As a result, this action can lead to weight gain. It is said that the more you understand about how emotions affect your eating habits, the better prepared you will be to overcome some of the obstacles you face in controlling your daily food intake.

Emotional eating refers to the act of eating to feel better. Most people see food as more than just a source of bodily energy. Sometimes, they enjoy eating, especially during their free time. There's nothing wrong with this habit. However, you should always know your limitations when it comes to food intake.

People often eat to deal with their bad feelings. However, this habit can lead to serious eating disorders, depression, obesity, and weight gain. If you don't want to experience any health problems due to excessive food intake, you need to find ways to solve this problem.

> ➢ *How to combat emotional cravings?*

Some people find it difficult to manage their emotions and eating habits. If you're one of them, you should always know the different strategies for managing your weight. For your guidance, here they are:

- Assess your level of hunger -
Before you start eating, assess your level of hunger. From 1 to 10, ten scales are the highest and it means you are full. If you notice that your hunger level is between 3 and 10, you need to avoid eating. You can only consume enough food if the hunger level is 1 or 2.

- Dealing with other comforting activities - Instead of eating more food while you're stressed, try to look for any alternative activities that can alleviate your current condition. Typical examples are listening to your favorite music, playing a musical instrument, chatting with friends or taking a walk.

- Practice Daily Exercise - It is undeniable that regular training can help reduce weight. But it can also help deal with anxiety and stress. Through daily exercise, you can avoid overeating. Therefore, you can easily manage your emotions as you develop your health condition.

- Use Three-Food Interference - This scheme is made by eating three types of nutritious foods first before eating your favorite foods. Typical healthy foods are vegetables, yogurt, fruits and many more.

As you can see, there are several ways to handle your emotions. Whether you're depressed or suffering from an emotional problem, you don't need to eat over and over again. Once you know how to handle your emotions, you won't be tempted to eat more food.

How to set objectives?

If you want to lose weight, you must set your ultimate goal. You also need to achieve your goals no matter what it costs. He says setting realistic goals before starting a weight loss plan has proven effective.

Sometimes people find it difficult to set weight loss and maintenance goals. Instead of worrying about this issue, accurate research is an ideal option. You can also seek help from trusted experts and friends for more details.

The precise steps for setting weight loss goals are not too complicated. Whether you are a beginner or not, you can easily make your own plan. For more details, here are some steps you should know:

Step 1: Start setting small daily goals - Before trying to lose more pounds, your first goal is to lose at least one pound each week. This is easier to achieve than reducing more weight in an instant. To make sure you achieve this goal, you have to establish your state of mind. You need to remind yourself about your goal of continuous daily workouts and a healthy lifestyle.

Step 2: Set Advanced Goals - Once you reach your first goal, you need to level up. For example, if you have already reached the goal of 30 minutes of walking per day, you should extend it to one hour of walking per day. You also need to eat smaller portions at each meal. For best results, you need to seek expert advice.

Step 3: Know your ultimate goal - If you want to have a perfect figure and body weight, you need to create ways to reach it. In addition to daily routines, you need to learn how to cook healthy foods, participate in fitness programs, and other related activities.

Step 4: Set deadlines for your goals
- If you notice that you are continually reaching your final goals, you have to reward yourself. Depending on your preferences, you can go shopping, go on a weekend trip, get a facial and much more.

Step 5: Stay Motivated - Although you've reached your primary goal, you need to exercise daily and live a healthy lifestyle. This can help maintain your body and weight the way you want.

When setting weight loss and maintenance goals, you should always be realistic. This means you don't need to write down any activities, especially when you really can't do them. During the first week of the weight loss program, make sure you can do it and that you have enough time to do any related exercises.

If you know how to set weight loss and maintenance goals, you don't have to worry about your daily activities. Since you need to write down all the activities you need to do, you will always be guided on how to reduce more weight.

   At the end of your exact goals, you don't need to ask your friends or other experts about the goal you really want to achieve. Therefore, it is easy for you to find ways to achieve your preferred goals.

Learning to eat...

Eating right doesn't mean you have to follow strict dietary plans. If you want to eat the right amount and type of foods, all you need to do is know the different foods that are loaded with perfect nutrients. You can do this by asking experts for help or reading health books.

> ### Adequate nutrition for weight loss

If you want to lose weight, you should concentrate on your daily meals. You need to know not only the foods you need to eat, but also the foods that can trigger your weight condition. Instead of worrying about it, here are some tips to keep in mind:

- Know the exact foods you need to eat - Some people abstain from eating to reduce their weight. This scheme is not advisable. If you're hungry, then you need to eat, but with limitations. If you continue to eat less food, you may suffer from complicated health problems such as fatigue.

- Eat more fresh vegetables and fruits - Nutritious foods can help you lose weight. These foods are perfect instead of eating unhealthy foods every day. If you change to a healthy lifestyle, expect to lose weight and have perfect body condition.

- Avoid skipping meals - If you keep skipping meals, you may be hungrier at the next meal. As much as possible, you need to eat five to six times a day. But, you have to eat a small amount. Never multitask and don't watch TV while eating. While you're eating, just sit down and pay attention to your food.

- Drink more water - Your body needs more water. Drinking more water is highly recommended than consuming soft drinks.

Before you eat, you have to drink a little

water to reduce your food intake. This can help reduce more body fat.

- Make a diary - Making a diary is an effective way to monitor your daily eating habits. Depending on your favorite foods, you need to write it down and you'll know the exact amount of food you eat.

- Try new foods - Even if you're planning to lose weight, it doesn't mean you have to forgo eating your favorite foods. Instead of eating the same kinds of foods over and over again, you need to try new, healthy recipes.

- Clean your kitchen - Means you need to remove all foods that can destroy your regular healthy diet. As much as possible, buy only a few foods suggested by your nutritionist. This is an excellent move to keep you from eating your favorite potato chips or other unhealthy foods.

Through your knowledge of how to eat well, you don't have to worry about your weight and body condition. You can easily motivate yourself to reduce more fat. If you are still confused about how to eat well, you are free to consult your nutritionist.

Note that there is nothing wrong with you eating food. Just make sure you're eating the right, healthy ones. You should also monitor your daily intake to avoid weight gain. If you are motivated and committed to your specific goal, you can achieve it no matter what it costs.

Alternatives to Weight Loss

To lose weight, some people prefer to buy supplements or pills. Others also wish to undergo various surgical procedures. Whatever choices you make, you need to be more informed about how they work.

If you want to rely on weight loss pills, you should examine each of the supplements available on the market. In some cases, people prefer to get expensive pills thinking they are more effective compared to cheap ones. Whether you choose affordable or expensive types, you can't easily determine their exact function if you don't understand their various ingredients.

Before buying any pill or supplement, the best option you should take is to start reading your reviews. When reading the comments, you have to navigate not just one, but several websites. The more reviews you read, the more likely you are to get more valuable information. To make sure you get an ideal type of weight-loss pill, it's best to seek expert help. You can also ask your doctors about the exact brand and type of pill you need to take.

Because money plays a vital role in buying effective weight loss pills, you don't need to rely on a very expensive one. In fact, there are several pills or supplements that are inexpensive, but come with effective results. Just be sure to compare one pill to another for a perfect purchase.

If you want to buy pills through local plans or online, be sure to browse your favorite store. Some stores are effective and some are not. To make sure you'll never be fooled by any scam provider, always read the different testimonials from your past and current customers. This can help you decide whether your desired store offers you an ideal supplement or not.

➤ *How effective is weight loss surgery?*

For those who can afford it, they prefer to rely on surgical procedures to remove excess body fat. If you are one of them, you have to find the best surgeon. The search for the best surgeon is not too difficult. You can find one by asking your trusted friends for help. You can also read some online comments to get a reliable surgeon.

Surgical weight-loss procedures are also effective. However, you must follow your surgeon's prescriptions before and after surgery. You also need to be more aware of your daily activities to avoid any side effects.

Whether you want to undergo surgical procedures, take pills, or practice the natural way of losing weight, you can get the results you prefer. Just make sure you know how to do it accurately to ensure positive results.

Conclusion

Do you have excess body fat? If the answer is yes, you probably have your own reason for choosing to burn more fat and achieve a perfect body weight condition. Why do people prefer to lose weight? An ideal body shape and a weight condition offer multiple benefits.

> ➢ *Other Weight Loss Benefits*

- Look Sexy and Attractive - If you keep asking why most people prefer to lose weight, most of them give similar answers. Both men and women want to reduce more body fat to make them more attractive.

- Look healthier and more active - If you're planning to lose weight, you need to eat nutritious foods like fruits and vegetables. As a result, you will achieve a perfect body shape while gaining the

benefit of practicing a healthy lifestyle.

- Save more money - When you're losing weight, you need to eat healthy foods. Therefore, you don't need to buy any food that can destroy your eating habits. This can help you save more money.

- Know how to manage your health condition - If you want to lose weight, you should probably start by consulting your doctor. Through this, you will learn several things about losing weight and living healthily.

With the various benefits of weight loss, everyone is encouraged to deal with reliable diet and training programs. Like others, you don't need to rely on multiple programs. Even if you keep participating in various activities, it will never be effective if you don't have self-control or motivation. Therefore, be sure to always follow your schedule to ensure effective results.

Weight loss control is not too complicated. If you have a specific goal, all you need to do is find ways to reach it. Through the help of weight loss management, you are guided to the specific activities you need to do. You will also know the different foods you need to eat.

For beginners, it can be difficult to follow their schedules. However, if you are anxious to reach your goal, everything will be fine. This is why most people prefer to lose weight using a special monitoring program.

Are you worried about your excess fat? If so, then you don't need to suffer its consequences. Don't let other people bully you just because of your physical appearance. If you are obese, then, you need to find ways to solve this by hand. Through the practice of a weight loss plan and management, everything will be in good condition. After several weeks and months, you will notice that you are losing

more fat.

Whether you want to lose weight or just maintain a healthy body shape, there's always a specific way to achieve that goal. After burning more fat, you have confidence to face other people. You are also free to wear the clothes you want.

By following these different guides, you are free to do whatever you want. So, start changing your daily activity now! Learn how to practice a healthy lifestyle and see how it affects your weight condition.

Looking and feeling good about yourself is possible. Although it may seem like a daunting task, with the right guidance, it will become much simpler. As long as you establish an effective routine and follow it daily, you will surely experience results. Don't be ashamed of yourself anymore! Start enjoying your life and start living a healthier lifestyle.

Now yes, I wish you the best in your

results, and remember, everything is practical; theory without action is of no use to you.

A big hug, your friend, Jessy!

By the way, when you achieve your results little by little, I highly recommend you, if you want to learn much more about methods of losing weight, my book, "Learn to maximize your metabolism", is a book that I'm sure will help you a lot on your path to "good health".

Without further ado, you can find it on the Amazon search engine, by title or by looking for my name, such as: "Jessy M. Brown"... Once again I wish you success in your results!